AN INTRODUCTION TO INTERMITTENT FASTING:

Losing Weight Without Sacrificing Your Favorite Foods!

J. L. Ceesay

Table of Contents

Introduction

What is Intermittent Fasting (IF)?

The word "Intermittent" is defined as "occurring in irregular intervals". The word fasting is an act in which one refrains from a certain activity for a specific period of time. Simply put Intermittent Fasting is refraining from food for a certain time period. IF has two components

- A fasting period: time interval in which you refrain from eating
- A feeding window: time interval in which you are allowed to eat.

What Intermittent Fasting (IF) is not?

- IF is not a magic wand for weight loss, you will not lose 10lbs in one week. You may however make consistent loss such as one pound per week.
- IF does not claim to be the best diet or the best approach to dieting for everyone. IF is a simplified diet method that works best for the busy individual.
- IF is not a necessity. IF, like every other diet is just a tool to help you lose weight. Think of it as another tool to add to your toolbox for weight loss. There are plenty of other additional ways to promote weight loss.

Why should you fast?

Intermittent fasting has many benefits, here are a few.

- Lower blood pressure
- Lower oxidative stress
- Increased fat burning
- Increased metabolic rate during the fast
- Improved appetite control

3

- Improved blood sugar control

- Improved cardiovascular function

Who is this manual for?

This manual is for those who:

- Want to learn the basics of intermittent fasting

- Want a to improve their health

- Want a consistent and manageable way to lose weight.

- Want to adhere to a diet but without the hassle of being limited to certain foods.

- This manual assumes that you have an exercise program to accompany an IF diet program.

Maximum fat loss cannot be achieved through diet alone. Instead fasting is a combination of exercise and diet that produces maximum fat loss. If you do not have an exercise program don't be discouraged. An exercise program can be as simple as jogging for thirty minutes a day. However, it should be noted that a well-designed training program that is tailored towards your goal will produce the best results.

Chapter One

How Intermittent Fasting Works

Intermittent fasting is a controlled pattern of fasting. Fasting? Meaning "not eat"? Yes. Most of us when we are hungry, we chow down on foods that we can grab. This includes junk foods, processed foods and most of the time, fast foods. Anywhere we go, we see fast food. Anywhere we go, we can find street food and so on. We eat three meals in a day and for most of us, three meals are not quite enough. We tend to eat more every time we feel hungry or every time we have a craving. Most of us know that we shouldn't give into every craving, but often we do. Regular meals are only supposed to be breakfast, lunch and dinner. Every other meal is just additional and most of the time not needed which causes us to add our weight and produce fat. If we are spending a significant amount of time engaged in physical activity then eating outside of regular meals should be alright. But if we do not do physical activity much, then we should resist these temptations.

So what do we do?

This is where intermittent fasting can be introduced into your routine. Eat all of the daily meals in a day and do fasting for the next twenty four hours. This doesn't necessarily mean that you cannot ingest anything at all. But limit your intake to water or any healthy drink including vegetable juice. But we recommend that water is better.

Water does a lot of good things in our body. It cleans our body and helps flush out unhealthy food. There are a lot of scientific studies and research that proves that intermittent fasting is very beneficial to our health. Remember, in the past our ancestors

5

did not have any fast food, junk food or street food whenever they are hungry. What do they do? They drink water in order for their hunger to be lost. Most of the time, we feel hunger not because we really are hungry but our body and mind just tells us to eat because it is what we're used to. We call this mental hunger. Sometimes, our minds can trick us. So this is a tip on intermittent fasting success. For example, today you can eat as much food as you like. But be prepared that after dinner tonight you are just allowed to drink water afterwards for twenty four hours. Drink water as much as you need to surpress your hunger. This process will train your body and mind to not let you eat when you do not need to eat. This fasting will eventually lead your body to use the stored fat and energy that has not been used for a long period of time. So you will lose weight and become healthier. Intermittent fasting is not advisable for all people. This is only good for individuals without health problems. Before you try intermittent fasting, you should first consult your doctor.

Chapter Two

Basic Dietary Guidelines

Will Intermittent Fasting Help You Lose Weight

Under certain circumstances, there is a great deal of evidence that says intermittent fasting can help with burning fat. Intermittent fasting is spacing your last meal of the day and your first meal the next day farther apart to as much as 16 hours. The rational is that after you eat, your body takes about six to eight hours to metabolize that glycogen, then to continue functioning it goes into your fat stores. But if we start feeding our body before that six to eight time period, or before the glycogen has been used, we never allow our system to tap into our fat storage. This makes it very difficult to ever lose weight. Of course we can go too far when we fast. When we go past a certain point, our system realizes it isn't going to get any more food and goes into starvation mode. At that point it basically stops using our excess fat.

Tests have shown that there are additional health benefits to intermittent fasting. These include increasing insulin sensitivity, reducing oxidative stress, and increasing the capacity for resisting cellular stress. All of these will retard aging of the cells as well as prevent diseases associated with cell damage. So is an intermittent fasting plan right for everyone? Actually, all of the factors that go into healthy weight reduction make it nearly impossible to find one magic potion that will be right for everyone. First, it is safe to say that pregnant women should never fast. A baby needs all the nutrients they can get, and some studies have actually suggested that fasting can alter the baby's heartbeat and breathing patterns, along with increasing gestational diabetes. Those that suffer from

7

hypoglycemia, a condition of abnormally lower level of blood sugar, should not go through periods of fasting. Your goal if you have this condition would be to normalize your blood sugar levels first, then if you decide to fast opt for a less rigid version of fasting. Those with diabetes also will not be helped with intermittent fasting.

You must realize that if you are going to fast, you must pay even more attention to your nutrition levels when you do eat. By continuing with a toxic-rich diet of highly processed foods, then proceeding to not eat for 15 or 16 hours, you could be doing your body more harm than good in the long run. Putting together a healthy diet plan to make sure you are getting the proper nutrition in the shorter time period you are eating in will be vital. Whenever you are going to make dramatic changes in your diet, even if they are healthy changes that will eventually greatly benefit your health, it may take a little while for your system to adjust to the change. But listen to what your body is telling you, and if you are going a little too ⬜uickly, don't fight it. Just go a bit slower with the changes, and if it is good for your system will eventually adapt. Tapping into fat storage is one of the secrets to weight loss. It not only re⬜uires good diet and exercise, but there is evidence that what you eat and timing when you eat is important.

Chapter Three

Why You Should Try Intermittent Fasting

Intermittent fasting is a controversial weight loss technique because it involves not eating food for an extended period of time. Many people have the notion that not eating will slow down your metabolism and send your body into starvation mode, but it turns out this is not true at all. In fact, the human body was designed to go long periods of time without eating, so intermittent fasting is actually a natural practice. Perhaps that is why it is so effective.

If you would like to lose weight but don't want to give up certain foods or don't want to partake in vigorous exercise, intermittent fasting is probably your best option. Fasting will help you lose weight quickly, even if you don't eat extremely healthy or exercise, although that would greatly enhance your results. This technique doesn't even require you to lower the amount of calories you consume. It simply takes a little bit of discipline in the beginning.

If you don't like the idea of fasting, perhaps the benefits will convince you to give it a try anyway. Intermittent fasting has many benefits that will greatly increase the quality of your life. Some of the benefits include:

- Rapid fat loss
- Lowered blood pressure and cholesterol
- Increase in energy, especially in the mornings
- Enhanced memory and cognitive ability

These are just a few of the many benefits that fasting can offer you. If you simply want to be a healthier and/or happier person, it would be of your best interest to begin an intermittent fasting routine. So, how can you begin?

There are a few ways one can begin fasting. One method, the one I prefer, is daily fasting. This involves eating your food for the day within a time period of 6 to 8 hours. This would mean you fast for 16 to 18 hours every day. The easiest way to do this is to skip breakfast in the mornings. You will benefit greatly from this. Even greater benefits will be experienced when you can lengthen the time spent fasting. For example, fast for 20 hours and eat for 4. Figure out what works best for you. Another method that also works well is weekly fasting. This would involve a period of fasting that lasts between 24 and 36 hours. So, for example, you would eat as you normally do for 6 days of the week, then one day you would not eat any food at all. Drink plenty of water during the time when you are not eating.

Intermittent Fasting - How to Do It Healthily and Safely

Intermittent fasting can improve health, reduce the risk of serious illness, and promote longevity. Perhaps you're intrigued and would like to give it a go but aren't sure how to start. Or maybe you have tried it once or twice and found it too challenging. This book will give you strategies and guidelines to practice intermittent fasting safely and successfully. There are three main ways to do intermittent fasting: a) only eat from 6pm to bedtime every day, b) a 24-hour fast on alternate days, or c) one or two 36-hour fasts each week. It's worth experimenting with all 3 strategies to see which works best for you in terms of your lifestyle and effect on your health and wellbeing. The guidelines I've given you below are mainly for the 36hr fast, but most are helpful for the 24hr fast as well.

Pick a day that isn't too hectic or demanding because you may experience some detox reactions. Make sure you have the option to relax if you need to. You will get more out of the experience if you make time to turn inward, still the mind, meditate, contemplate, and listen to your inner guidance. Enlist support from people close to you before you start. It's great to fast with your partner so you can both motivate each other and share experiences. Eat lightly the evening before by choosing a large salad or steamed vegetables with some lean protein. There is no point gorging the night before because it will make you feel even hungrier whilst you fast. It's best to avoid alcohol as well. Keep hydrated during the fast as your body has an essential need for fluid. Water, herbal teas, and vegetable juices are good choices. Have at least 2 liters of fluid during the day. Avoid coffee, tea, carbonated drinks, fruit juice, and alcohol. Have 1 or 2 glasses of vegetable juice as it will provide important electrolytes as well as having a health-boosting alkalizing effect. Try juicing celery, cucumber, chicory, fennel, and watercress. Avoid carrots and beets as they are □uite high in sugar.

About fat loss supplements

They don't work. Yep, fat loss supplements are a huge waste of money. They don't speed up your metabolism or anything. In fact most of them just suppress your appetite so you eat less. Appetite suppression is something you can control with sheer will power so why pay money for it?

Engage in light exercise such as walking, stretching, and gentle yoga. This is not the day to do an intense gym workout or anything too vigorous. Add some breathing exercises such as yogic pranayama. A few minutes of practice offer amazing benefits from detoxification to boosting energy. Expect some detox symptoms such as headaches, feeling groggy, or short periods of feeling jittery. These are made worse if you usually have lots of caffeine and sugar in your diet. Avoid taking over-the-counter medication to reduce these side effects. Instead rest, go for a walk, and practice breathing exercises. Listen to your body wisdom and if you feel unwell or it gets too much then have some food. Your body knows best. Break the fast gently the following morning. Have water or herb tea and a piece of fruit when you get up then 30 minutes later have your usual breakfast. Eat as usual for the rest of the day (you probably won't feel the need to overeat). Enjoy the changes in how you feel during and after the fast. Notice changes in your energy, emotions, and mental state. You may notice food is far more enjoyable on the day after the fast because your senses are heightened. Recognise that it can take a few attempts to get used to this practice. After a few weeks your body will get used to it and the benefits you feel will increase as the discomfort simultaneously decreases.

The essentials for a successful intermittent fasting program

- Dedication
- Determination
- Your body
- A good exercise program

What you don't need

- You will not need to buy specific foods, eat what you want to but remember moderation is the key factor.

- You will not need a personal trainer if you are well-versed in training. If you are not you may seek out a trainer or look online for information.

- You don't need any suspect fat burning supplements.

Chapter Four

The Wonderful Benefits of Intermittent Fasting

The pattern of eating called "Intermittent Fasting" usually means one fasts for a period of time and eats for a period of time. Many choose a 24 hour cycle of fasting, then eat healthy the next day, and continue this process as a lifestyle change. Research has been done on animals to find the benefits of this type of fasting, and you will be happy to know it really can be beneficial to your health! Intermittent fasting can add 40%-56% more years to your life! That in itself is reason enough to do it.

However, other benefits include body weight reduction and fat oxidation. When you fast your body is forced to scavenge for fuel thus removing aged and damaged cells in the process. This sort of cleanses the body of undesirable and unwanted things and helps the weight loss and benefits of the good food choices be increased and more beneficial to your body. Rats have been shown to have long-term and improved survival after heart failure after being on an IF eating plan. Researchers are also saying that it might help age related deficits in cognitive function, too, so that tells me that it might help ward off Alzheimer's Disease and other types of Dementia!

Your risk of heart disease and other heart ailments may also be decreased when you start a healthy intermittent fasting regimen. Your risk for other chronic illnesses and diseases will also most likely be reduced. A healthier you can begin with intermittent fasting and healthy food choices. Keep carbs to 50-100 grams per day. Many women eat between 1200-1500 calories per day, and when limiting their carbs, they are still losing weight. Men can handle up to 2000 calories per day. Of course, less is best, and you need to determine caloric intake based on your activity such as working hard and exercising. Drink lots of fluids, especially water and exercise in the evenings if possible. This will help with those late night cravings. Once you start eating and drinking healthier, your body won't crave as much (if any) junk food, so making healthy food choices will simply get easier and easier as you progress in the intermittent fasting routine. Alternate Day Fasting or ADF means alternating days of eating and not eating any food, but there is also an intermittent fasting called Modified Fasting where you consume about 20% of your normal calories one day and then eat normally (but healthy) the next day. This is often more attainable for people because they feel less deprived when they are able to at least eat something daily, and it still has most of the benefits of the ADF regimen. Whatever you choose to do, make sure you tell your health care professional of your plans so he or she is aware and can work with you to reach your goals. If you want to lose weight, lose fat and feel better, then intermittent fasting might be the answer for you!

One of the hormones in your body is called IGF-1 (insulin-like growth factor 1); it helps your cells grow and is particularly important in growing children. As you reach adulthood, however, it decreases significantly. This is important, since as you grow older it appears to have adverse effects: it accelerates aging and can even lead to cancer. So it's not something you want high levels of when you're older. And studies have shown that intermittent fasting decreases it.

Also, in your brain is a protein referred to as BDNF (brain-derived neurotrophic factor). It is important because it has been shown to help stem cells turn into new neurons. This takes place in a section of the brain called the hippocampus, which is critical in relation to memory and learning, BDNF has many effects: it appears to protect against dementia and Alzheimer's disease, and it also acts as an anti-depressant, suppressing anxiety.

15

Intermittent fasting also helps increase autophagy, which is a system in the cells that gets rid of damaged molecules that could lead to serious neurological diseases.

Diabetes

Diabetes comes in two forms: diabetes I and diabetes II. We will be mainly concerned with diabetes II. As we saw earlier, all cells use glucose as fuel. But it can't get into the cells without insulin. Insulin is produced in the pancreas according to the amount of glucose in the blood; it's role is to allow the glucose to enter the cell. Most of the cells in your body have what are called insulin receptors that bind to insulin that is circulating in your blood. When a cell has insulin attached to its surface it allows glucose in, so it obviously plays an important role in your body. But too much can be detrimental. Insulin increases your hunger, promotes the storage of fat cells, and it has been linked to diabetes and heart problems. One of the major problems associated with insulin is what is called insulin resistance. In this case the pancreas produces insulin, but insulin receptors on the cells no longer work properly, and don't allow glucose to enter as they should. With no place to go, the glucose continues to circulate in the blood, and the cells soon begin to starve. The body realizes that something is wrong and the pancreas produces more insulin in an attempt to get sucrose into the cells, but this causes the pancreas to overwork, and it eventually begins to wear out. The result is diabetes II.

Studies have shown that intermittent fasting improves your insulin sensitivity. This in turn allows your body to do a better job of controlling your blood glucose levels after meals, and therefore helps rest your pancreas. Both of these are important in relation to the prevention of diabetes II.

Rules for Fasting

- It is best to use a 5 - 2 approach, with regular meals 5 days a week, and two days of restricted food (500 calories for women, 600 for men).
- Stay hydrated. Drink Plenty of water; it helps flush out toxins.
- When not on fasting days (and even when fasting), keep your nutrition maximized. In particular, eat sufficient vegetables, fruits and whole grains.
- Remember that 12 hours of fasting is needed for the effect. From 12 to 18 hours is best. It plateaus beyond 18.
- You can exercise during fasting periods, but don't overdo it.
- Be careful of fasting if you are diabetic.

Chapter Five

The Truth About Fasting

The benefits of fasting have been big news lately. But how effective is it? Most people are interested in it as a weight loss tool, and indeed you can lose weight using it, but in reality it has many benefits beyond weight loss, and some of them are ⬚uite miraculous. It has been known for many years that it extends the life of mice, worms and flies rather dramatically, and even appears to extend the life of monkeys. Does it extend the life of humans? Many people are convinced that it does, but the truth is that we're still not sure, although it looks hopeful. There's no doubt, however, that it has health benefits in relation to heart disease, cancer, dementia, and even your mood and well-being. It can't be called a cure, but it does set the stage for healing by allowing vital parts of your body to rest and recuperate. There's no doubt that excess eating puts a burden on your body, and that it needs an occasional rest. Indeed, studies have shown that if it doesn't rest, it forgoes much of the repair and regeneration needed for optimal health.

Glucose, Glycogen and Fat

Your body needs energy to run properly, and it gets this energy from the food you eat. Food is turned a form of sugar called glucose. Your cells (and particularly the ones in your brain) need a constant supply of glucose, and if it gets low you begin to feel fatigued and weak.

Glucose circulates in your blood after you eat, and it is used up fairly rapidly as you go about your everyday tasks. If not replenished, it is, in fact, depleted in a few hours. This creates a problem: how do you maintain a good supply? Glucose itself can't be stored,

18

but it can be turned into a form called glycogen that can be stored in your muscles and liver. From here it can be drawn out and used as needed. It is usually good for about 10 to 12 hours. What happens when it is depleted? The body then turns to the fat cells that are stored throughout your body. They can be broken down and converted to what is called ketones. This is, of course, what dieters look for, namely, the loss of fat cells. But you have to be careful if you remain in this stage for too long. The body soon begins to break down protein; it can also be converted to glucose through a rather complicated process. And this causes the loss of muscle - something you don't want. Indeed, in most diets, a fair amount of the weight loss comes from muscle loss along with depletion of water (leaving you dehydrated). So don't be deceived.

Weight Loss Through Fasting

As it was mentioned earlier, you can lose weight by fasting, but most doctors and dieticians do not recommend long fasting periods because they can have an adverse effect on your overall health. In addition, it is difficult for most people to fast for long periods of time. A better alternative is what is called intermittent fasting in which you fast on certain days of the week, and eat normally on the others. One form of this is alternate-day fasting. In this case you fast (or restrict your calories) on one day and eat normally the next. This works well for some people but Dr. Michael Mosley of BBC has put forward what he calls the 5-2 fasting diet. In this diet you restrict your calories only two days a week. He suggests 500 calories for women on these days and 600 for men. This is much easier for most people to do, and it appears to give the same results as more extended fasts.

19

How does weight loss occur?

Weight loss is a process of being in a caloric deficit. A caloric deficit is when you use more calories than you are consuming. Weight loss cannot occur without a caloric deficit. Go back and read the last sentence until you have fully grasped the concept of weight loss.

What if I want to gain weight?

Since weight loss occurs when we are not consuming enough calories to meet our daily use, then weight gain is the opposite. Weight gain occurs when we exceed our daily caloric needs thus the extra calories are stored as fat. If you induce a stimulus such as weight training, then the extra calories will be used to repair and improve the damaged muscles thus enlarging your muscles and ultimately results in your gaining muscle weight.

Preserving Muscle

You always hear people saying "I want to lose weight" or "I need to lose some weight" but they never specify what type of weight. Muscle contributes to your total bodyweight too, so does water, and your organs and so on. You could lose 10lbs of muscle, but would you be satisfied? The correct phrase is "I want to lose fat". Typically fat (adipose tissue) is what most people are referring to when they want to lose weight. However, what inevitable happens during a diet is muscle loss.

Here's why.

Muscles are calorically expensive. Think of it as a bank. Say each pound of lean muscle requires 25 calories to uphold. So if 100lbs of your total bodyweight is pure muscle than you need to eat 2,500 calories a day just to maintain your muscle mass. Say now you want to go on a diet so you reduce your calories down 2,300. Now a problem arises. You don't have enough calories to maintain your muscle mass. Still using the bank analogy, you are now presented with two choices you can sell off your muscle (break down muscle tissue to pay for the other muscles and reduce total spending) or you can take out a loan (break down fatty tissue for extra calories). Ideally you want the latter because that's what fat is for, right? Fat is to be used as energy when we are in a deficit.

So then how does muscle loss occur? Muscle loss occurs when we exceed our loan limit. Say our deficit is now 1500 calories and we still need 2500 calories each day. We find ourselves down 1000 calories however we can only take out a max loan of 500 calories from our fat reserves. This limit occurs because there is a limit to which fat can be broken down. Thus we are force to breakdown some of our muscle to pay for the rest. So in conclusion to minimize muscle losses always reduce your daily calorie needs by small increments (200 or 100 calories) so that you don't exceed

your loan limit. Utilize a strength training program to ensure that your body realizes that your muscles are needed.

Are all calories e□ual?

Yes, are calories are equal. There is no such thing as good food and bad food just food that are more calorie dense (higher in calories) and food that are lower in calories. If you still have doubts about a calorie being a calorie, go read <u>about the professor who lost 27 pounds while eating only Twinkies.</u>

All calories are equal, but are all foods eꞁual?

These chemicals are potentially harmful and thus should be avoided or kept to a minimum. As a general rule the closer the food is to its natural form, the better. I am not saying that you can't enjoy your favorite foods but simply stating that the majority of your diet should consist of natural foods. The benefits of a healthy diet are endless but here are a few

- Higher energy levels
- Better mood
- Less risk of diseases
- Stronger immune system
- Healthier skin
- Stronger bones
- Longer life

Macronutrients and Caloric Maintenance

I won't delve too much into this topic as there is a wealth of information on the internet and it would be outside the scope of this manual. So consider this a brief introduction to macronutrients.

Macronutrients are protein, carbohydrates, and lipids (fats).

Protein: If you are a serious weight lifter or an athlete then you should be aware of the importance of protein. Proteins are the building blocks of muscle and aid in recovery after a training session. Of the three (carbs, fats, and protein) protein is the most important. Protein can be found in meats, dairy, nuts, and legumes (beans). The general rule for any athlete is 1 gram of protein per pound of bodyweight. For example, if you weigh 150lbs than you should strive to eat 150 grams of protein per day. Each gram of protein is equivalent to approximately 4 calories.

Carbohydrates: Carbohydrates are your body's main source of energy. The majority of your daily calories will come in the form of carbohydrates. Carbohydrates come in two major forms, sugars and starches. Sugars are easily digested and thus enter the blood stream immediately. Starches take a while to digest and are often stored in the muscles as glycogen. Each gram of carbohydrate is equivalent to approximately 4 calories. Examples of carbohydrates are bread, pasta, grain, sugar, potatoes, and rice.

Fats: The media has completely destroyed the reputation of fats and thus when we hear the word we often associate it with synonyms such as "bad". However fats are not all bad and some fat is necessary for optimal health. There are three types of fats, saturated, unsaturated and trans. Generally, trans-fat are bad and increase your risk of heart disease. Saturated fats are not necessary bad but should be limited to a small percent of your diet. Foods with saturated fats are meat, butter, lard, cream, etc.

Unsaturated fats have been proven to decrease your risk of developing heart disease. You can include unsaturated fats into your diet by consuming foods such as avocados, nuts and any food cooked with olive oil.

Caloric Maintenance: caloric maintenance is simply the number of calories your body needs in day to maintain homeostasis, which is to have no weight gain or weight loss but to stay at equilibrium. Caloric maintenance varies with each individual. It may be higher if you are younger, more active, and have more muscle mass. Your caloric maintenance will be achieved through a combination of protein, carbohydrates and fats. Generally for new trainees I recommend a standard 40/40/20 ratio which means 40% protein, 40% carbohydrates and 20% fats. For example I generally eat around 3000 calories a day to maintain my bodyweight. So, 40% of 3000 is 1200 calories. 1200 divided by 4 is 300 grams of protein. If I followed a 40/40/20 ratio then my diet would be the following.

3000 calories (40/40/20)	Protein 40%	Carbohydrates 40%	Fats 20%
calories	1200	1200	600
grams	300g	300g	67g

It should be noted that consuming 300grams of protein in one day is next to impossible as that would mean you would have to chug down copious amounts of protein shakes.

24

Thus a more realistic macronutrient ratio would be a 20/60/20 ratio. See below for an example.

3000 calories (20/60/20)	Protein 20%	Carbohydrates 60%	Fats 20%
calories	600	1800	600
grams	150g	450g	67g

To determine your caloric maintenance a good starting point would be to use a daily calorie calculator. You can find many calorie calculators online such as the one at Freedieting.com. My suggestion is to use the calculator to obtain an estimate. Then test the estimate for two weeks if you happen to gain weight subtract a little, such as 200 calories from the estimate and retest for another two weeks. If you lose weight than try adding 200 calories to the estimate and keep testing until you find your caloric maintenance.

However the good news is that with enough experience you will eventually be able to accurately guess how much calorie certain foods consume. For example I am now able to eye-ball foods and obtain a good estimate of how many calories were in the meal I ate.

Starvation vs. Hunger

A common mistake to make during a diet is to confuse hunger with starvation. People will often feel their stomach growling and assume that if they don't eat soon they will vaporize into thin air. Well I was kidding about the vaporizing, but people will often prematurely end their fast because their stomach was rumbling. The premise is that once your body enters starvation mode your metabolism rate drops thus you will burn fewer calories and your diet will be in vain. However, that is not the case. Studies on fasting and metabolism has shown that the earliest sign of a decrease in metabolism occurs after 60 hours and none of the IF programs will have you fasting more than 24 hours so you won't have to worry about a reduced metabolism. So, what do I do about the hunger pangs? From personal experience I found that if you just ignore them and continue about your day the hunger will go away immediately. However do not mistake hunger with physical pain. If your stomach is in physical pain and actually hurts then you are doing something wrong. Please consult a physician.

An interesting phenomenon that I learned about hunger is that you are able to control it. Before I started using intermittent fasting I used to eat 6 meals a day. You know the whole "if you eat more you will increase your metabolism nonsense" which has been proven wrong in case you were wondering. During my six meals a day diet I normally ate at 8:00am. 11:00am, 2:00pm, 5:00pm, 8:00pm and 11:00pm. So, during the first week of intermittent fasting I would become hungry around the same times because my body was so used to eating at those times. However, I ignored my hunger and by my third week of IF my feelings of hunger were slowly dissipating and I could go longer without eating. Not only that but I would only feel hungry during the feeding window of my intermittent fasting program. So what's the moral of the story? You are in the master of your hunger.

Conclusion

Back during the ice age era our ancestors would go days without eating. They lived their life not knowing when their next meal would be or what it will come from.

So our body is well-adapted for survival. This is why our body stores fat, to have an extra storage of calories when we are starving. Fat is our insurance. Another reason why our body prefers breakdown our muscle is that it sees that it can reduce daily spending by getting rid of the calorie expensive things such as muscle.

However our ancestors didn't have to worry about losing muscle because their lifestyle was more active. They had to run, jump, climb trees, scale mountains, throw spears, carry the old and wounded, and so on. So their body's top priority was to keep their muscle or else they wouldn't survive in such a world.

Fast forward to today and a majority of us lead sedentary lifestyles. Our body says "oh it's okay for us to get rid of these muscles, it's not like we use it for anything". That's where weight training comes in. Weight training gives our body a reason to keep our hard-earned muscles. Add weight training and healthy eating to your IF diet to achieve maximum health benefits and weight loss success.

Legal & Disclaimer